Disclaimer:

Stephen Rader is not liable for any injuries or damages that individuals might incur by attempting to perform any of the exercises or feats of strength depicted or discussed in this book. Any individual attempting to does so at their own risk. Consult with your physician before beginning an exercise regimen.

Acknowledgments

I'd like to thank my wife, Patricia, for serving as my editor and, most of all, for supporting me on this journey to become a personal trainer at such an advanced age. I'd like to thank my daughter, Sophia, for serving as chief photographer and graphic designer and for creating all the exercise images in this book. I'd also like to thank my son, George, for inspiring me with his own personal calisthenics journey and for compelling me to try and keep up with him.

Table of Contents

Introduction 1
Who Is the Target Audience? 3
What Is Needed to Get Started? 4
What Is Covered In This Book? 4
What Will You Gain from This Book? 5
My Perspective and Purpose 6
Definitions 7
    Sets and Reps 7
    Workouts, Micro-Workouts, and Splits 7
    Rest 8
    Strength Starting Points and Strength Potential 9
    The Volume and Intensity Continuum 10
The Exercises 13
    Warm Up 13
    The Push Group 14
        Push-Ups 14
            Incline Push-Ups 15
            Regular Push-Ups 16
            Decline Push-Ups 16
            Diamond Push-Ups 17
            Archer Push-Ups 18
        Dips 19
    The Pull Group 21
        Rows 22
        Pull-Ups 24
        Chin-Ups 24
    The Squat Group 25
        Assisted Two-Legged Squat 26
        Unassisted Two-Legged Squat 27
        Bulgarian Split Squat 28
        Hover Lunge 29
        Pistol Squat 30
The Program 31
    Phase 1 31
    Phase 2 32
    Phase 3 34
Sample Workout Log 37
Additional Resources 39

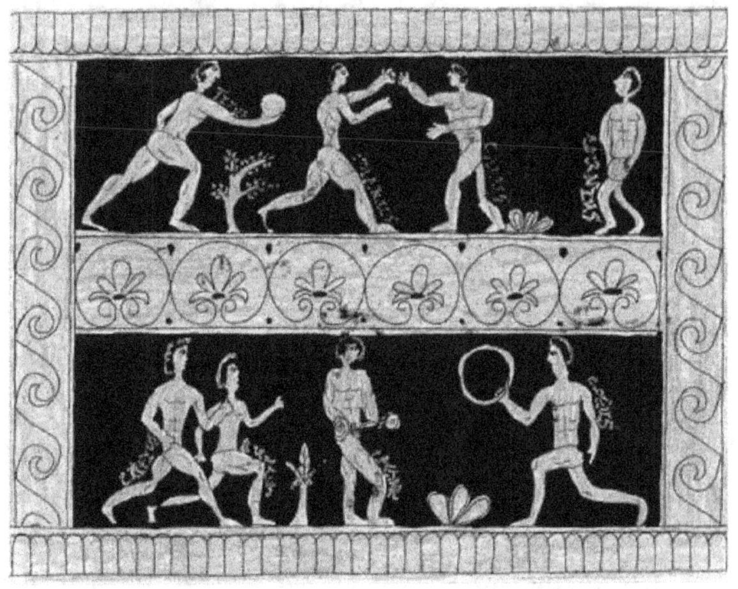

INTRODUCTION

Welcome to calisthenics, the most versatile, approachable, and effective form of strength training you can do! You are in good company; calisthenics has helped people get fit and strong for thousands of years. Calisthenics was "invented" by the Greeks several thousand years ago. They named it, developed it, and perfected it, as they did with most things worth knowing, doing, and having. Kalli (good, beautiful) sthenos (strength). They definitely used it to their advantage in times of battle. This book is about strength training using body-weight calisthenics. This means that we are not using any external weight to provide resistance as is done in weightlifting. Rather, we are using our own body weight as resistance and are relying on variations in body position and limb placement to make exercises more or less difficult.

This book is designed to help you get started or move to the next level in calisthenics and to develop or improve a progressive program of your own that can offer a lifetime's worth of strength training and personal development. The comprehensive three-phase program included here can be done by anyone, from the absolute beginner to the more experienced athlete. We will be doing body-weight calisthenics, which means that we will not be adding any external weight for resistance. Instead, increased resistance is accomplished by changing the body position or angle, and these leverage changes will make the exercises more or less difficult.

For this calisthenics program, we will utilize three different exercise groupings, the Push Group, the Pull Group, and the Squat Group. This will give us a firm foundation upon which to build our strength and abilities. We will begin by mastering the basic movement patterns until we are comfortable performing them multiple times with good form. We will then build a basic workout program and learn to progress in volume and intensity. Strength gains will follow rapidly. Once we have progressed in volume and intensity, we have set the scene to move to more advanced exercises and re-program our workouts for the next phase.

Who Is the Target Audience?

The target audience for this book is people who are new to strength training, or are interested in trying calisthenics for the first time regardless of their strength-training background, or have been doing calisthenics for a while but need a strategy to move to the next level. Recovering weightlifters? You are welcome here. Exhausted chronic cardio junkies, come on inside! If you are out of shape and stressed about it, but even more stressed about how to get started and what to do, this book is for you. If you have been doing push-ups for a while now but need to know where to go next, this book is for you. Calisthenics in general and this program specifically will appeal to people who are not necessarily interested in gyms, equipment, and a lot of time and hassle around exercising. The exercises described here can be performed just about anywhere with minimal to no requirements in terms of equipment, money, time, and special clothing.

What Is Needed to Get Started?

Aside from willingness and an open mind, the only thing needed in terms of equipment to get started is something to use for the pulling movements that will be described later. This can be a bar or set of gymnastics rings or suspension grips that can be moved to about waist height or higher and can safely support at least half your body weight. As will be explained in more detail later, you can use just about anything, including a table-top, two dog leashes connected to one another and hung over a limb, a tree limb, or two chairs placed back-to-back with a sturdy stick across the top.

What is Covered in This Book?

This book will describe the three essential movement groups that are required for balanced, full-body strength and conditioning: the Pull Group, the Push Group, and the Squat Group. The book will teach you several different exercises within each of these three groups, how to perform them correctly, and how to change them slightly in order to make them more difficult. You will learn how to set your starting point by picking the exercises that are appropriate for your level in the three groupings, and you will learn how to: master the basic movements (Phase 1), program your workouts to make continuous progress (Phase 2), and finally, move on to more difficult exercises and reduce your reps and then build them up again (Phase 3).

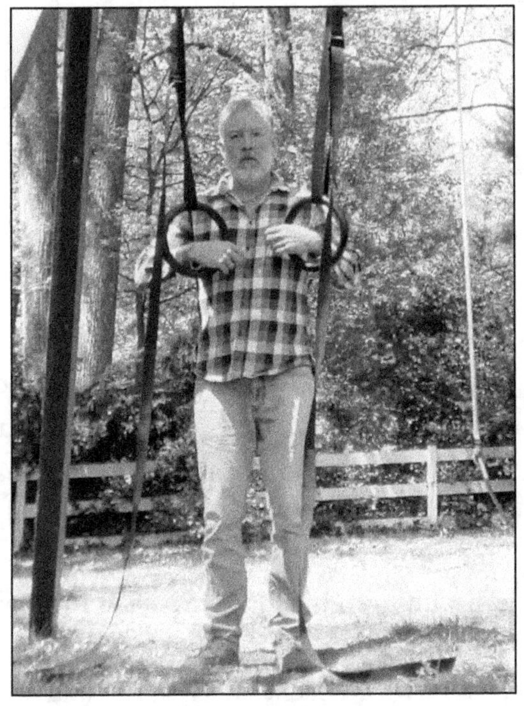

Gymnastics rings

What Will You Gain from This Book?

Most importantly, you will gain strength, fitness, flexibility, a tighter core, and a new sense of autonomy and independence about strength training. You will gain the skills and knowledge for a lifetime of approachable and enjoyable growth and improvement! You will gain an enthusiasm for simplicity in exercise and the excitement that comes with learning that you need nothing much more than a floor or a tree branch, a few minutes a day, and a creative mind to get a good workout. And I would like nothing more than if you got from this book a confidence and understanding of how you might achieve a strength goal that you never before thought possible. I've met many people both younger than me and older than me who have said "I have never been able to do a pull-up." Well, let's get that first pull-up!

My Perspective and Purpose

I am a certified Progressive Calisthenics Instructor and I see two main facets to my job: to educate and continuously motivate clients and students to learn that anyone can do strength training and make continuous progress, and to de-mystify and untangle the concept of fitness and health from the massive web of disinformation and profit-driven dogma that pervade the fitness industry. I am your very own coach, cheerleader, and BS-buster! This book represents an entry-point to this world.

DEFINITIONS

Sets and Reps

For any strength training exercise, calisthenics or otherwise, if you perform the movement once, you have done a single repetition, or rep. Performing several reps in a row is a set. If you do 10 push-ups and then rest and then do 10 more, you have done two sets of 10 reps. "Drop and give me twenty" means you have done one set of 20 reps.

Workouts, Micro-Workouts, and Splits

It used to be the case that a "workout" was always a single block of time during the day dedicated to exercise. During that block of time you may work all the muscles of your body or you may "split" your work into related exercises for only a part of the body. If you do all your pushing sets, all your pulling sets, and all your squatting sets in a single 40-minute period of time, for example, you have done a full-body workout. If you are more advanced or have less time, you may "split" your workouts into pushing and pulling movements one day and squats on the next. This is an upper-body / lower-body split routine. Similarly, if you do all the push exercises on one day, all the pull exercises the next day, and all leg exercises the third, you have done a push/pull/legs split.

Regardless of how you may group your exercises (or not), these days "micro-workouts" are becoming popular. Micro-workouts allow you to break up the workout throughout the day so that you are not performing all your exercises in one session. You may do pushing exercises in the morning, pulling exercises in the early afternoon, and squats in the evening. (You wouldn't want to do the same kind of exercise more than once a day.) With this method you don't need as much time at each session, and will be less likely to feel the need to change clothes and drive somewhere to do your workout. Calisthenics and micro-workouts go very well together. For beginners, this book will guide you through a full-body workout three times a week. You can do the workout all at once or in micro-workout fashion, whichever you prefer.

Rest

Rest can refer to the time between sets (measured in seconds or minutes) or the time between performing the same workout or group of movements (measured in days). Both are important, but I'm not a fan of timing things and I AM a fan of simplicity, so generally speaking, the rest between sets can be the time it takes for your breathing to begin to return to a normal rate or a little longer. This is usually around a minute to 90 seconds. The shorter the rest between sets, the more intense and exhausting the workout. In terms of rest between workouts, as a beginner it is best not to perform exercises from the same group more than once a day or on consecutive days. If I do push-ups today, I would not want to do them again tomorrow. I should note, however, that this venerable notion that rest is necessary and days off between working the same muscle group is a subject of some debate. As a rule of thumb, if you feel fresh and ready, you have rested enough, and if you feel sore and tired and unmotivated, you have not.

Strength Starting Points and Strength Potential
There is a wide range of strength starting points and strength potential among people. There are those of us who may be able to do pull-ups even if we do not practice them regularly. On the other hand, there are others for whom pull-ups will always be very challenging if not impossible. And yet those same people may be able to do three or four times as many squats in a set as I can. Some people will master dips quickly and others will not. That is exactly why this book presents a range of exercises within each grouping, with the easiest being something that just about anyone can try, and the most difficult likely being near or beyond the range of what some people would consider trying. Regardless of your experience, your genetic potential, and your ambition, there is a large variety of exercise choices available to you in this book.

The Volume and Intensity Continuum

In strength-building, there are two very important concepts: volume and intensity. The overall amount of exercise that you do in a given period of time is referred to as volume. This is the total number of sets and reps in your workouts and the total number of days per week where you are exercising. Intensity refers to how hard you work within a single set or how difficult each set is in a workout. Let's say that you are able to do 25 push-ups in a row with good form, and after 25 you can't do another. By the end of the 25th rep, you have reached "muscular failure." No matter how hard you try, you cannot get a 26th rep. Taking your sets regularly to muscular failure is very intense and challenging to the body and mind. If, however, you did sets of 12 or 15 reps per set, you are stopping well short of muscular failure. When you do this, you can do multiple such sets in a workout before exhausting yourself. You are able to perform a higher volume of push-ups than if you took each set to or close to muscular failure. You cannot perform a high volume of high intensity sets. This concept is important when you are figuring out just how hard you should work in your sets and your workouts. You need to work hard to make progress but not so hard that your workouts are grueling and you dread them and cannot recover enough to be ready to do them again in a day or two. The guy slowly pedaling an exercise bike while half-heartedly curling a 3 lb. dumbbell while talking on the phone is wasting his time. On the other hand, the guy who spends all his energy trying to get eight reps on bench press with 185 lb. on his second set of the day (like me in 1985) likely won't be able to complete his workout and make any progress. You need to figure out how hard to work in order to make progress but not quickly exhaust your physical and mental energy. My general rule is to take each set just past the point of it becoming difficult and burning my muscles, but several reps short of muscular failure. When I do this, I know I will be able to do at least two more such sets of the same exercise in this workout. I will take the third and final set closer to failure. This is exactly what we will be doing in Phase 2 of this program.

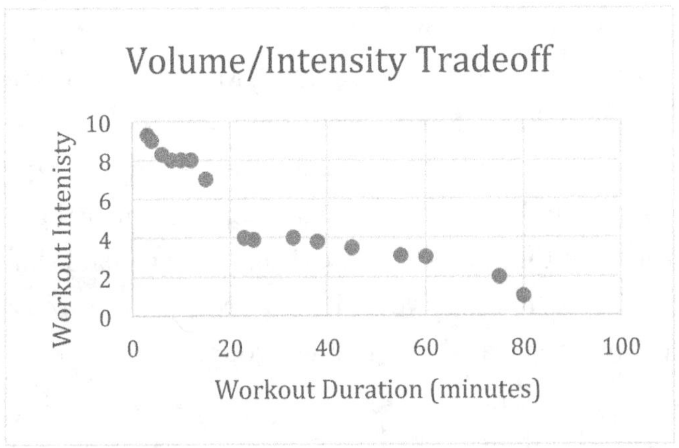

Volume and intensity are not opposites, but rather lie on opposite ends of a continuum

Process and Goals

The fitness world of today will have you immediately setting specific goals and then measuring your progress towards them, as if this is all that is important. I need to lose 15 lbs. by summer or get 15 pull-ups by the end of July. But an obsession with specific goals and measuring objective progress obscures the satisfaction and value that you can receive from focusing mainly on the process itself. For example, I think it's safe to say that many people who became obsessed with getting visible abs, and then eventually do so, may end up questioning the point of the whole thing. The reason is that they were obsessed with one body part and mainly how it looks, and had to devote a great deal of effort and self-control to getting that specific little visual effect (that requires a bare midsection to even see!), where they could have been focusing on their overall health and strength. Maybe it's more important to enjoy your physical fitness and the quest to master a particular exercise, and more so, the desire to get up tomorrow and do it all over again. Specific goals have their place, but they pale in comparison to the general goal of getting up each day of your life and working towards a stronger and more capable version of yourself.

Ok, let's get this thing started!

THE EXERCISES

Core

A strong core is absolutely fundamental to the exercises in this book. However, I am not including any specific core exercises in the programs. The exercises included in this book are the ones that I consider to be the absolute basics for strength and health. A strong, tight core is essential to performing these exercises and, even better, your core strength will grow through the proper performance of the exercises described in this book as your overall strength grows throughout this program.

Warm Up

You can take a fairly intuitive approach to warming up. I don't need you to do 15 minutes on the treadmill at x% of your heart rate max, but I do need you to see the value of getting into the groove before pushing yourself too hard, and appreciate the danger of jumping up off the couch and attempting your personal record of pull-ups while cold, for example. You might want to warm up with some active stretching and a slow rep or three of each of the exercises you will be performing in your workout. Get the blood moving and the muscles engaged in what they're about to be asked to do. And importantly, get your mind focused and the distractions set aside.

> *Group 1 – Push* – The Push group involves the muscles of the chest, shoulders and triceps (the back of the arms) and includes variations of push-ups and dips.

PUSH GROUP EXERCISES

Push-Ups – The baseline push-up is performed with your toes and hands both on a level surface. The back and neck remain straight and the core and glutes tight and engaged. Your elbows should be tucked in towards your sides rather than flared out such that, if viewed from above, you would look like and arrow rather than a T. Your hands should be about shoulder width apart. The wider your hand position, the easier the movement (but the more troublesome it can be for your shoulder health). Lower yourself slowly to the ground so that your nose nearly touches, and then push yourself all the way back up until your arms are straight (this is the "lock-out" position). Elevating your upper body will make the push-up easier (performed against the back of a couch, for example) whereas elevating your lower body will make it more difficult. It can also be made more difficult with a close together hand position ("diamond" push-ups) or leaning your body weight towards one arm or the other ("archer" push-ups). Diamonds and archers are both intermediate exercises. Choose a variation of the movement that allows for at least six and no more than 12 repetitions per set with good form (but don't worry too much about the numbers).

Incline Push-Ups – this is the easiest push-up variation. Elevate your upper-body to reduce the amount of weight that you are pushing. The higher your upper body, the easier the push-up.

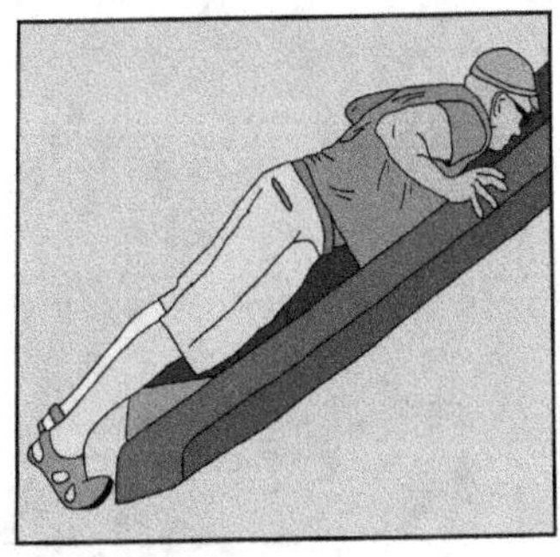

The starting position of the incline push-up

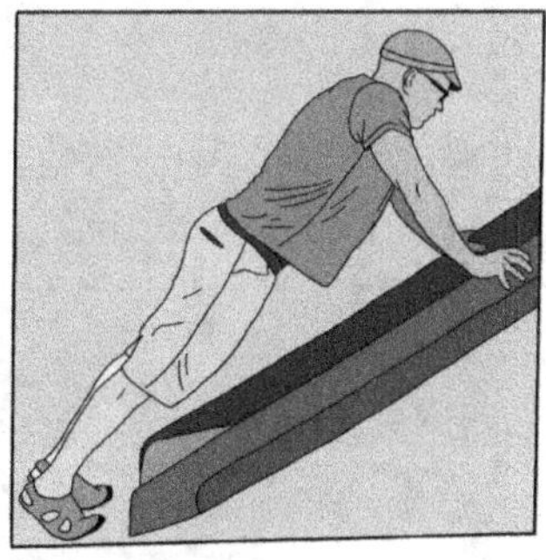

The ending position of the incline push-up

Regular Push-Ups – hands and toes are both on a flat surface, elbows in towards the sides rather than flared out.

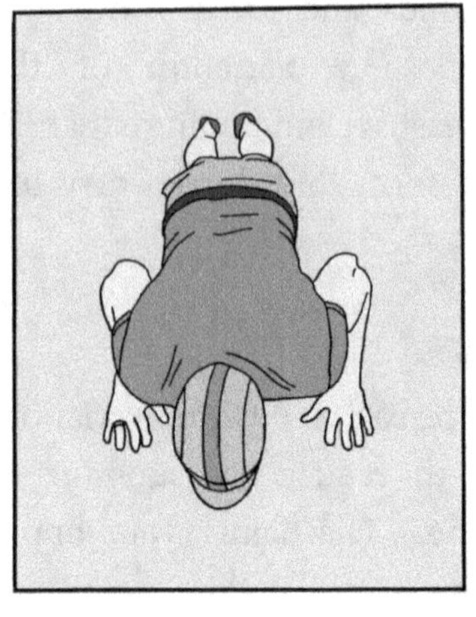

Regular push-up start position

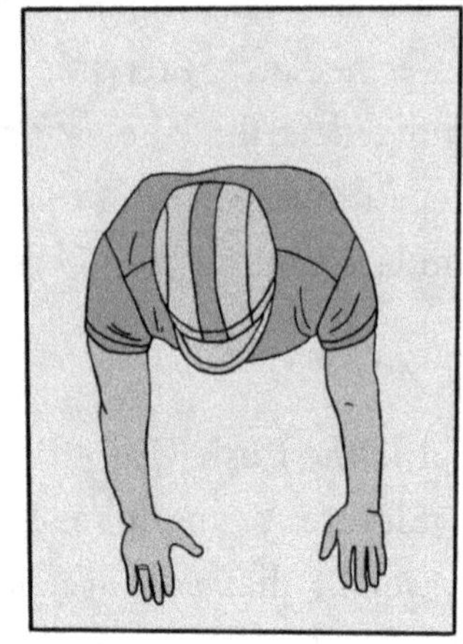

Regular push-up end position

Decline Push-Ups – elevating your feet places more weight on your upper body, making the exercise more difficult.

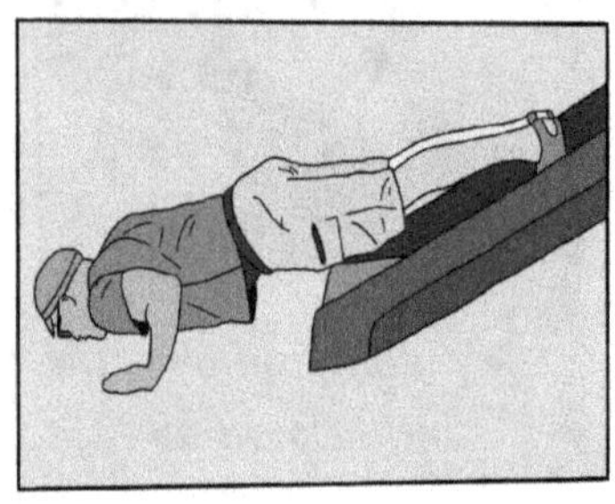

The starting position of the decline push-up

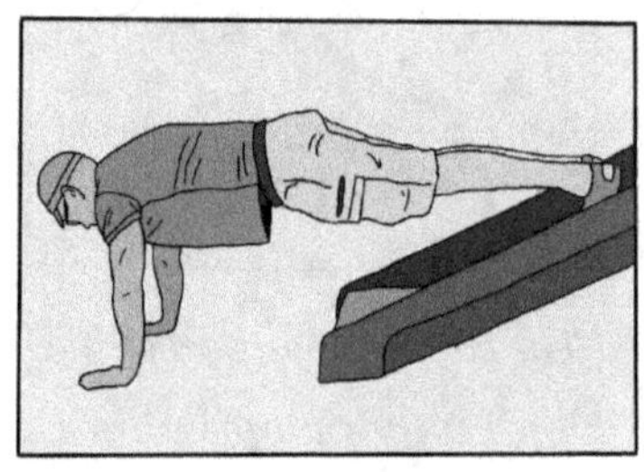

The ending position of the decline push-up

Diamond Push-Ups – so named because your hands are positioned so that your thumbs and index fingers form a diamond, this is a difficult exercise. The hand position concentrates the weight and makes the move more challenging and also targets your triceps.

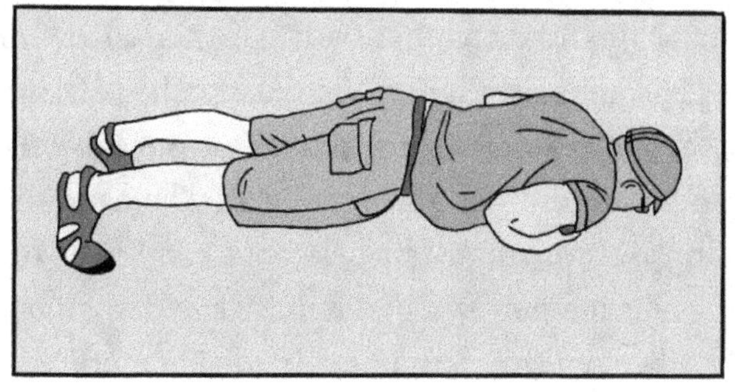

Diamond push-up start position

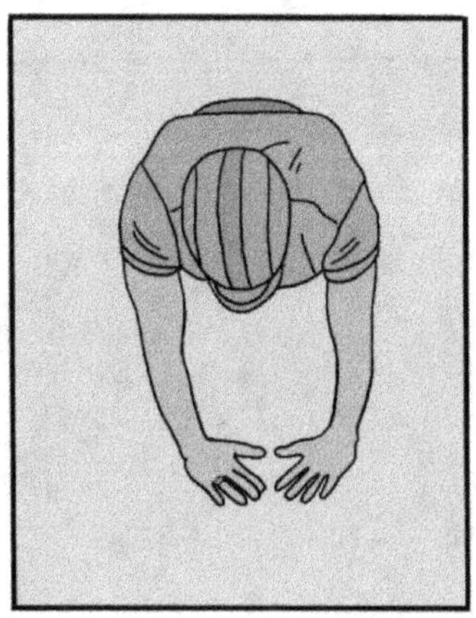

Diamond push-up end position

Archer Push-Ups - these are one of the most difficult variations of push-ups, as you are altering your body position so that you are concentrating most of your weight on one arm. Archer push-ups should not be attempted until you have mastered all the preceding variations listed in this book. They are called "archer" because your posture if viewed from above would resemble that of an archer with bow and arrow drawn back. The more straight your outstretched or support arm, the more weight is distributed to your pushing arm and the more difficult the exercise is. The hand of your pushing arm will almost be below the center line of your body. You can perform the exercise by alternating arms every other rep (in a kind of side-to-side motion) or do one arm at a time.

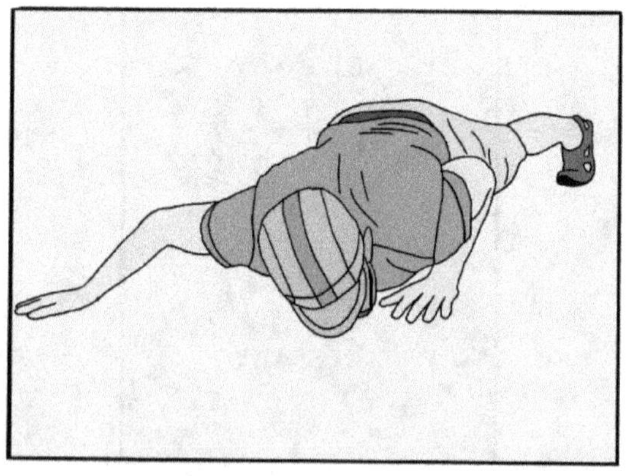

The archer push-up start position

Dips – Dips are a more difficult push exercise because you are pushing your entire body weight. They also require some kind of equipment, such as a set of parallel bars or suspension grips or gymnastics rings that are about waist-height. You grasp a bar or ring in each hand and then push yourself up to the lockout position and then lower yourself down again until the upper arm is parallel to the ground. If there were a small body of water below you, you would be "dipping" your toe in the water at the lower position. Dips make you very strong but there are many fewer body posture changes available to you with this exercise, and so dips are much more difficult than push-ups to progress without adding external weight.

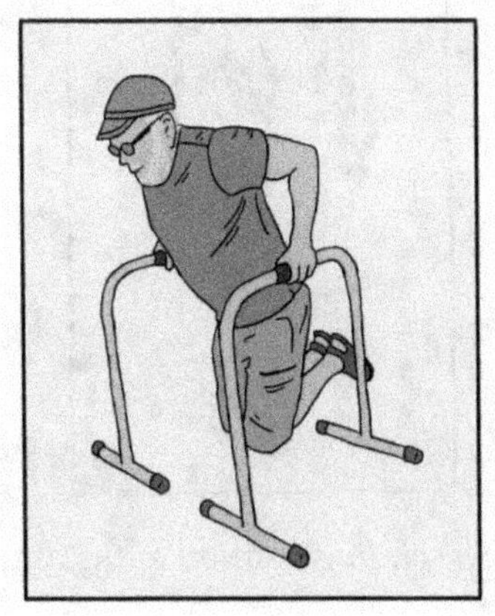

The starting position for the dip

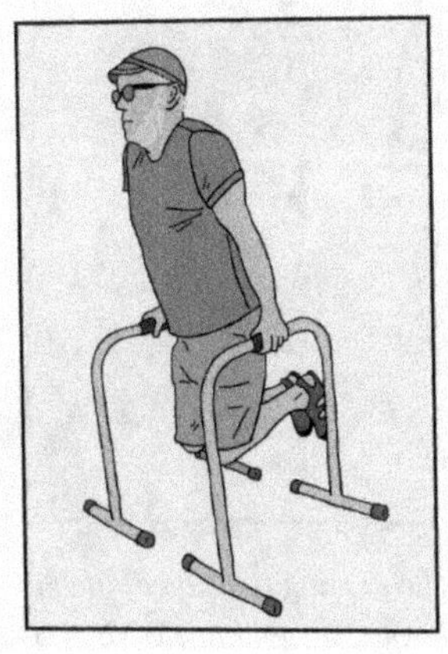

The ending position for the dip

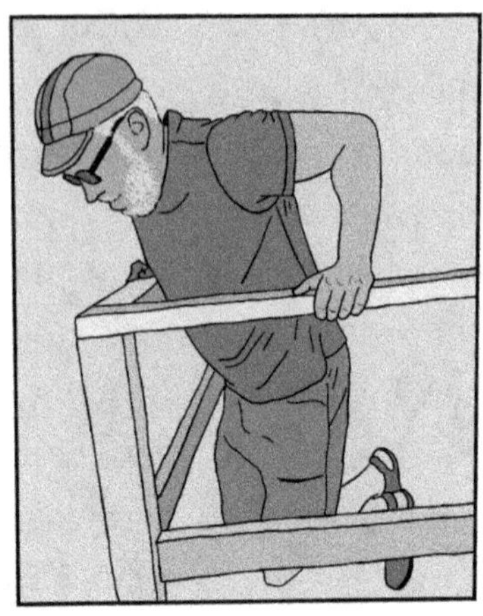

A fence can be a great dipping station. Dips can also be done at the point where two kitchen counter-tops meet

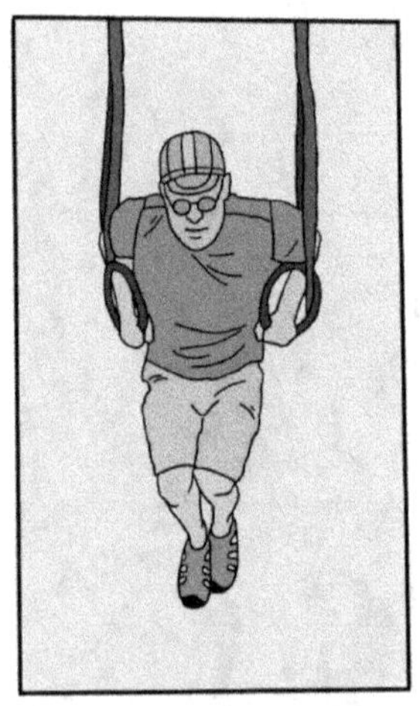

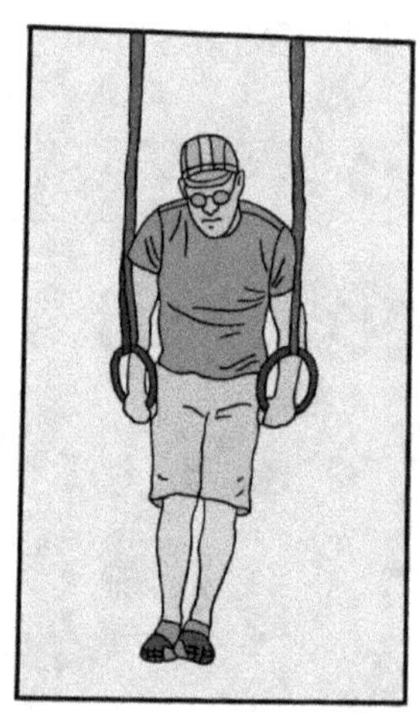

The starting position of the dip performed on gymnastics rings. Dips on gymnastics rings are much more difficult than dips on a stable object like a fence.

The ending position of the dip

Push Group Exercise Selection - If you are a beginner, start with push-ups. If you are an absolute beginner, start with incline push-ups. However, if you are strong enough to do at least 12 reps of the regular push-up and can do at least a few of some of the more advanced push-up variations, then you have the choice of progressing to even more difficult push-up variations OR dips OR both. It's up to you. Dips build solid strength because you are lifting your entire body, but they do require an external object such as dip bars or a fence. Push-ups require only the floor. You can experiment with your pushing exercises, just make sure that you are consistent in your workouts and track your progress in some way.

Group 2 – Pull – the pull group involves the muscles of the back and biceps and includes variations of rows and pull-ups. Both exercises require a bar or object that is suspended above the ground that you can grasp and pull yourself up on. This can be a pull-up bar, a tree branch, a table top, a fence, or a set gymnastics rings, for example.

PULL GROUP EXERCISES

Row - The row is performed on a bar or object at roughly waist height, and the feet remain planted on the ground during the movement. It is called a row because it is the movement you perform while seated in a boat with a set of oars in your hands. The row is like the opposite of the push up. Position yourself under the bar and grab it with hands roughly at shoulder width apart. If you extend your body straight out below the bar such that your legs are fully extended and heels are planted on the ground and toes are pointed to the sky, then this is the most difficult version of the movement without using another piece of equipment. Bending your knees so that your feet are flat on the ground makes it easier. A higher bar makes it easier still. Pull yourself towards the bar until your chest touches it, pause, and slowly lower yourself back down to the lockout (arms straight) position.

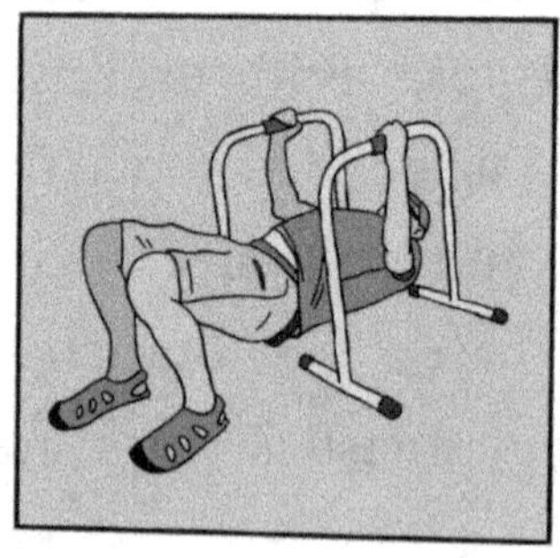

Bottom position of a row using a "neutral" grip, with palms facing each other

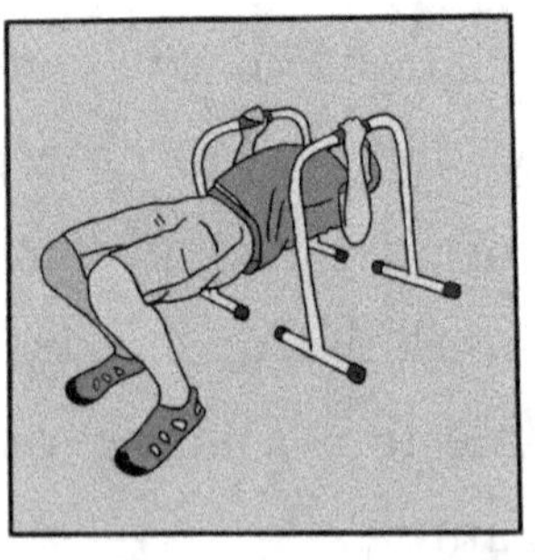

Top position of the row

In the absence of a bar or set of rings you can use a table top for rows. This is quite handy, but make sure it is a sturdy table that will not tip or rock or fall on you. A card table or a smaller table with a round top would not work well for this purpose.

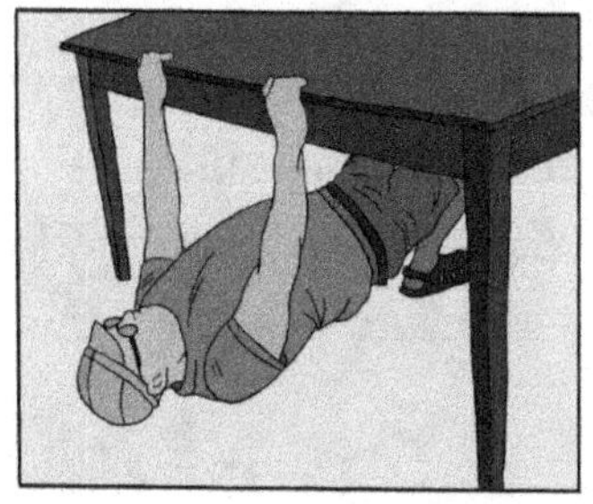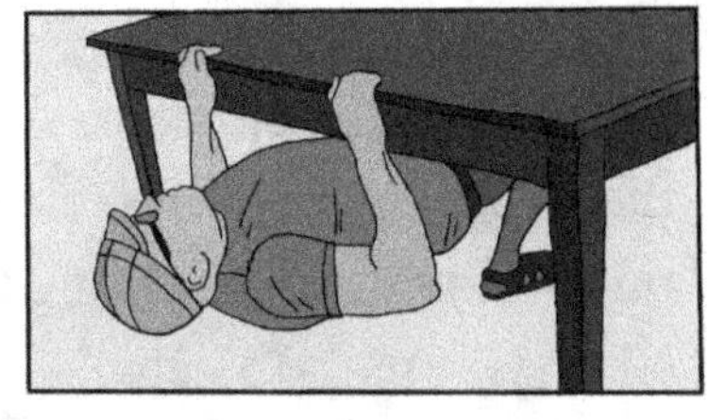

Dining room table rows

You can also use two dog leashes. Four-foot-long dog leashes connected at the clasp can be tossed over a tree limb or an overhead support. Wind duct tape around the handles for a more forgiving grip.

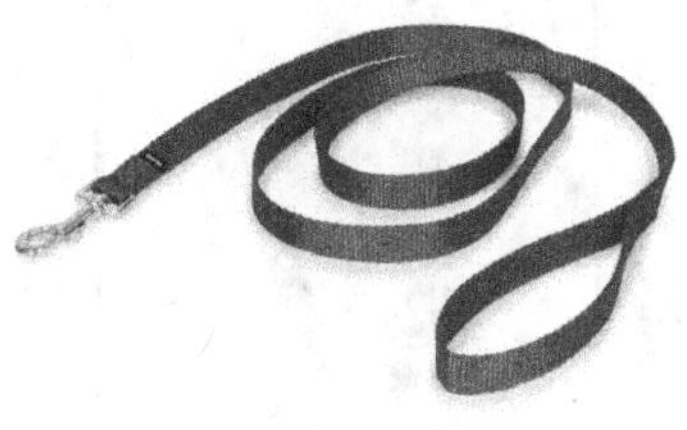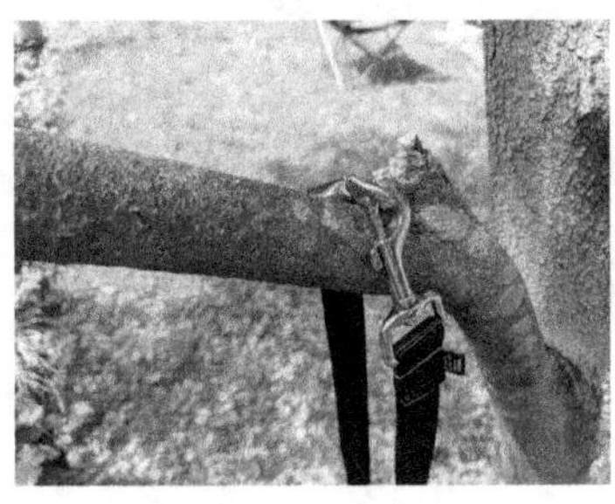

Pull-Up – the pull up is performed on an overhead bar, limb, or set of rings or trainers. This is a very difficult movement that requires you to lift your entire body weight. The pull-up is performed with the palms of the hands facing forward. Make sure to extend your arms all the way at the bottom of the movement and keep your body straight throughout.

Chin-Up – the chin-up is a version of the pull-up with the palms toward your face. It is slightly easier than pull-ups with palms facing forward, and puts a bit more emphasis on the biceps.

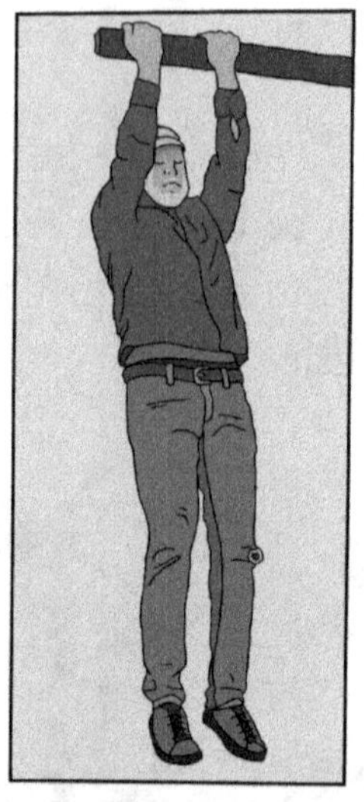

The starting position of the chin-up

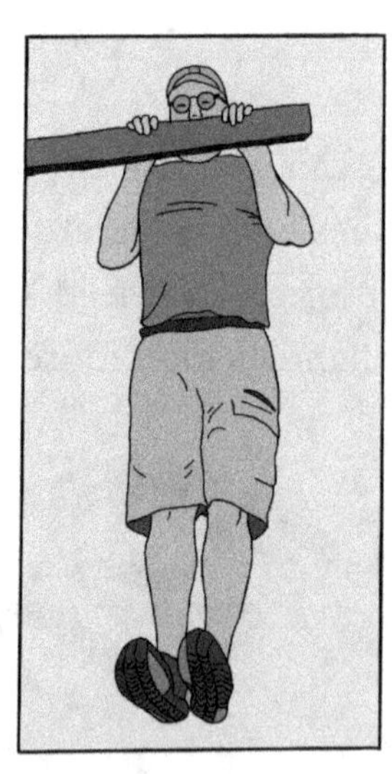

The ending position of the pull up

Group 3 – Squat - The squat is a basic human movement that children do naturally but without practice is lost by most people as we get older. In terms of overall strength requirements, the squat is probably the easiest of the three movements discussed in this book, because after you master the form you will be able to perform many reps. However, the squat is the most technically challenging of the three movements because a proper squat requires quite a bit of balance as well as flexibility and mobility in the ankles, knees and hips. It is best to practice the basic movement until you've mastered the form before adding reps. Understand that almost all of the "squats" that you see people performing in videos and in popular media are really only partial movements. If you squat down far enough that the angle formed by your lower and upper leg is 90 degrees, this is parallel. Unless the thighs are below parallel to the ground at the bottom of the movement it is not a full squat. Performed properly, your rear end should almost touch the backs of your ankles. Almost all of the difficulty of the squat is found in the bottom half of the range of motion, which is why the partial squats that I see most people doing are of far less value than a squat with full range of motion. The squat can be made much more difficult by moving it to one leg.

SQUAT GROUP EXERCISES

Assisted Two-Legged Squat - You can start re-learning the squat by facing a pole or edge of a door. Hold on to the door as you squat down. At first, squat only as low as your knees and ankles will allow, but hold the movement for as long as you can. If you have pain do not go any further. Slowly practice going down further and further until your thighs are below parallel to the ground. Once you are comfortable with this, you can begin to let go of the bar or door. At first you will need to shift your upper-body weight forward to avoid falling back.

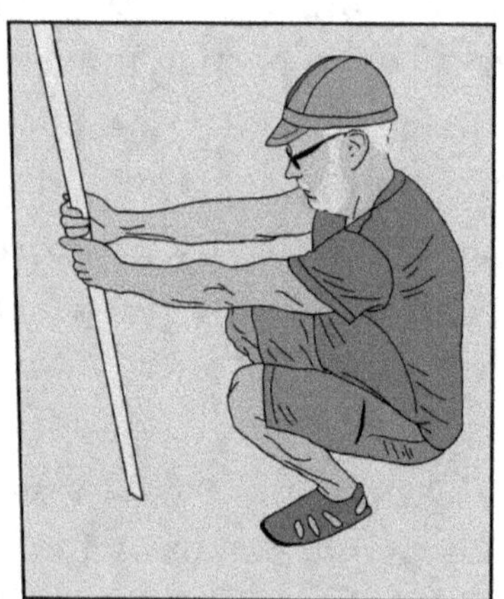

Pole-assisted squat

Unassisted Two-Legged Squat – same as above but take away the pole. After you are comfortable with the full range of movement using assistance, you can slowly remove your hands from the assisting object. You will need to get used to shifting your bodyweight forward to keep your balance. Another method is to slowly walk your hands up and down the pole as you squat, gripping it lightly rather than grasping it and holding tightly. You are using it as a guide and support if you have any balance issues. You may also want to perform your squat without assistance but then use the pole when standing back up or simply to stabilize yourself. Once you are ready to perform the squats unassisted, you will find that your reps build up rapidly. Nevertheless, it is always good to stay familiar with the single-rep movement and reinforce your range of motion as often as you can. It's also beneficial to get into the bottom position and hold it as long as you can.

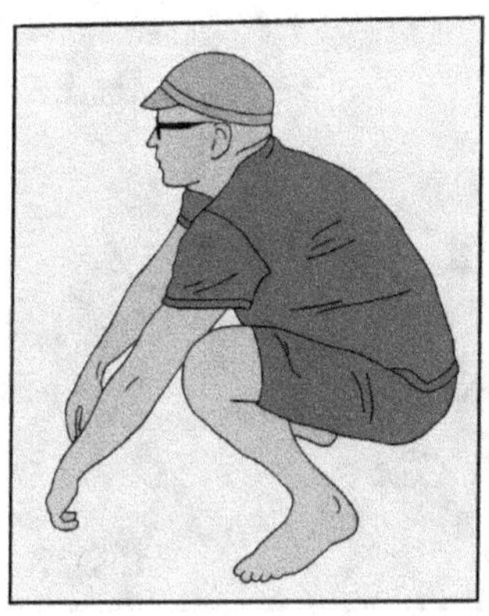

Unassisted squat

Bulgarian Split Squat – The Bulgarian Split Squat is the easiest of the single-leg squat variations. Such unilateral exercises are very beneficial for overall balance and to address muscular imbalances, such as your left leg being weaker than your right. Stand with a stair or stool behind you and place the non-squatting leg back, resting the tops of your toes on the stair or stool. If you are not used to it, this exercise will challenge your balance, so you may want to have something in front of you that you can use to stabilize yourself as you squat. Squat down so that your upper leg is at least parallel to the ground and then return to the starting position.

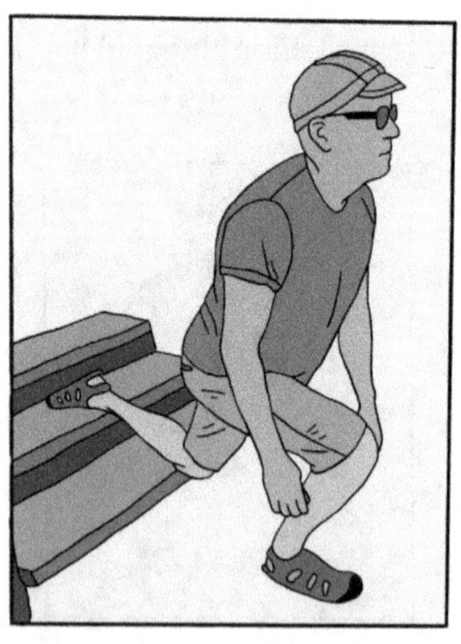

The Bulgarian Split Squat

Assisted Hover Lunge – the hover lunge is a bit like the Bulgarian split squat without the object behind you that you rest your foot on. The non-squatting leg is still behind you but is not touching anything. This makes the exercise more difficult as you must lift the entire weight of the non-squatting leg. Without assistance this exercise requires good balance and strength. It may be useful to stabilize yourself with something in front of you to put your hands on until you are strong and balanced enough to perform the movement without assistance.

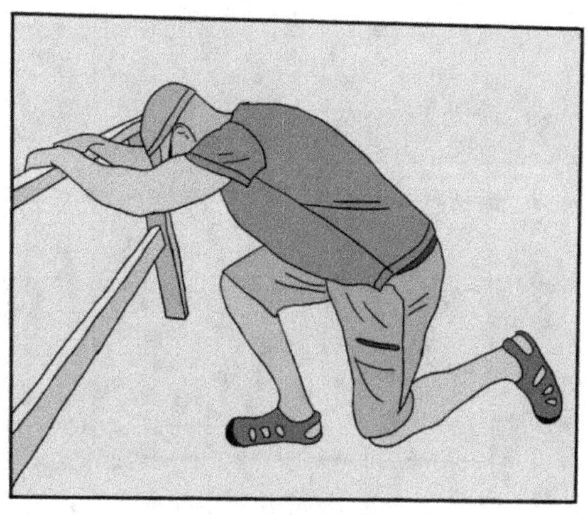

Assisted hover lunge

Assisted Pistol Squat – The Pistol Squat is the king of all single leg squat exercises. In this case, the non-squatting leg is held in front of you and as you squat down, it is extended out so that it is parallel to the ground at the bottom of the movement. When done properly in the squatted position your body shape resembles a pistol. This is an advanced movement and requires a lot of strength, flexibility, and balance in both legs to do the squat itself and to hold the other leg up and straight. A doorway or a set of rings or trainers can be used for assistance.

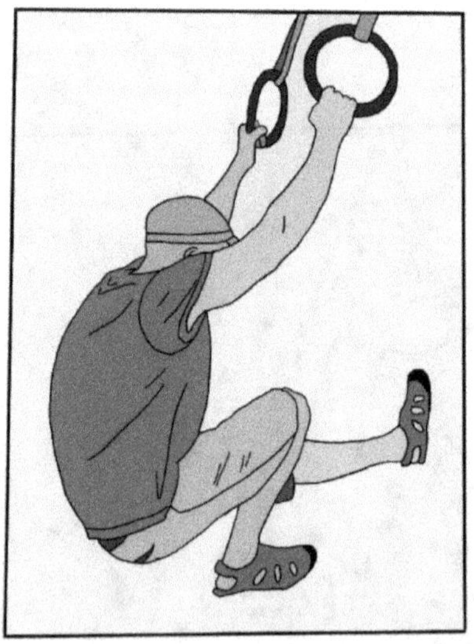

Assisted pistol squat

THE PROGRAM

PHASE ONE

Objective - Phase 1 involves mastering the exercises using strict form and full range of motion so that they are comfortable to you and you can perform them with good technique. In Phase 1, you will not worry about sets, reps or workouts. You won't worry about numbers at all. Instead, you regard Phase 1 as practice or learning the movements. You will practice the moves as much as you can without exhausting yourself.

Programming - You may wish to try the Grease the Groove method. This method involves practicing the movement pattern at very low reps frequently throughout the day in order to get better at it (which they like to call "reinforcing the neuro-muscular pathways"). Let's say that you want to perform regular push-ups for your pushing movement for this program, but you can only do three with good form. We want to get to at least 6, so try doing sets of two or even one throughout the day, as often as your strength and energy levels will allow. You need not be systematic or count the total number of sets. You might, for example, do a push-up every time you pass through your bedroom doorway. Because you are not exhausting your muscles using this method, you are able to perform the movement frequently while your neuro-muscular system learns the movement and the pathways are strengthened.

Stay in Phase 1 for as long as you need to in order to be able to perform a set of at least 6 reps of the three movements you would like to do for your workouts. How long this takes depends on your starting point, but you will certainly see marked progress in a week if not a few days. You can skip Phase 1 if you are already there. Once you are able to perform at least six reps of each of the three exercises, you are ready to move on to Phase 2.

PHASE TWO

Objective - In Phase 2, we will program your workout, and then progressively increase your volume (and therefore your strength). This will feel like a standard workout with volume and frequency. We will use a progression method outlined in the book Grind Style Calisthenics by Matthew Schifferle.

Programming - After a good warmup, we will perform three sets of each exercise, keeping track of how many reps were performed. Rest only as long as you need to between sets. If we performed the same number of reps in each of the three sets, in the next workout we will try to add a rep (with good form) to the first set. In subsequent workouts, we will "back fill" reps to sets two and three, trying to bring them up to set one. After this has been accomplished, we will start the process over by adding a rep to set one. It might look something like this:

Monday: 10, 10, 10
Wednesday: 11, 10, 10
Friday: 11, 11, 10
Monday: 11, 11, 11
Wednesday: 12, 11, 10
Friday: 12, 12, 11

This back-filling method is very effective because it prevents you from exhausting yourself on the first set and saves a little strength for the latter sets where you can make progress.

A beginner workout for Phase 2 might look something like this:

- Incline (chest elevated) push-ups
- Knees bent rows
- Pole assisted squats

Establish your 3 set baseline as a starting point and then record your sets and reps using the sample workout log included with this book and shown below. Once you have reached three sets of 12 reps per exercise without a breakdown in form, it is time to move on to Phase 3. (Note, 12 is a rather arbitrary number. There is a lot of dogma attached to "rep ranges" and what they might mean for strength, muscle growth, and conditioning. I don't really buy much of this, and generally feel that higher rep ranges are better, particularly as you age, because they mean that you are not under enough of a load to cause joint pain. You may adjust your target rep range higher or lower if you prefer, just always keep in mind that you need to be working hard in each set rather than chasing numbers. Go by feel more than count.)

PHASE THREE

Objective - Once you have made it this far, you have progressed through a set of exercises by adding good reps consistently. Congratulations, you are stronger! In Phase 3, we will now choose the next most difficult exercises in the three groupings and start the process over again. Because these are more difficult exercises than the ones you performed in Phase 2, you will not be able to do as many reps as your totals in that Phase. You will first need to get good at the movement so that your form is on point. Then you will be ready to start your first workout in Phase 3, where you will likely be getting six or seven reps in your first set.

If in Phases 1 and 2 you did incline push-ups, knees bent rows, and pole assisted squats, it might be time to move on to:

- regular push-ups
- legs straight rows (heels on the ground)
- unassisted squats

If, however, you started with regular push-ups, straight leg rows and regular squats, then in Phase 3 you can progress to:

- feet elevated push-ups or diamond push-ups,
- feet elevated rows (you can use a stool, a chair or a bucket, for example)
- Bulgarian Split Squats

Programming - Start with three sets of maximum reps with good form and then add a rep using the Grind Style technique until you have reached three sets of twelve reps per exercise. Note that you can apply this three-Phase program to any level. For example, if you have "graduated" from push-ups, rows and squats, you can start over with dips, pull-ups and assisted single leg squats.

If you keep at, before you know it you'll be doing handstand push-ups, muscle ups and pistol squats!

So………. Let's do this thing!

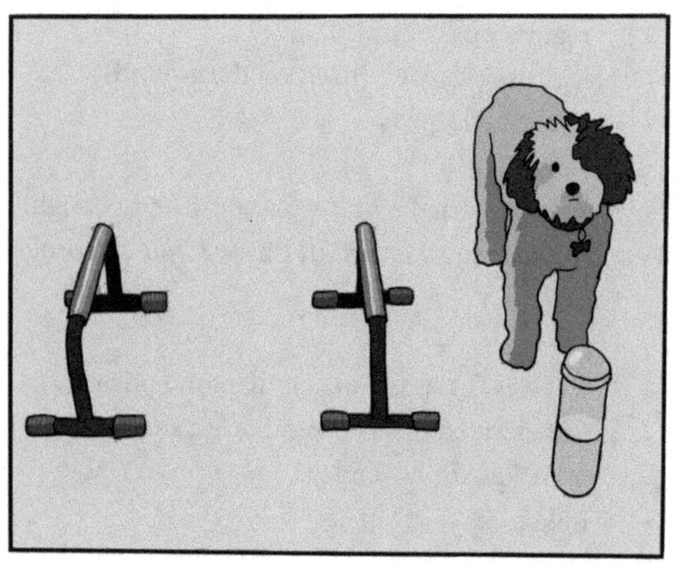

This athlete needs no equipment

SAMPLE WORKOUT LOG

Accompanying this book is a sample workout log in Microsoft Excel format, a portion of which is shown below. *Using a log such as this is entirely optional,* but I do recommend recording your sets and reps somewhere. You begin to keep track when you start Phase 2 and throughout the rest of your training. If you prefer paper and pencil, you may also print this and use it as a paper copy. The attached file includes four weeks of training for Phase 2 and four weeks of training for Phase 3 (on its own tab). Shown below on day 1 are the items you need to enter yourself. The totals will be computed automatically if you are using the Excel version of the log. Additionally, in the progress column, you will see an asterisk (*) for any total that exceeds the total for the same exercise on the prior workout. This is also done automatically and indicates that you have progressed.

I have entered sample data below so you can see how the programming works. Once you have entered the rep counts for each of the three sets, the rest is automatic.

Week	Day	Date	Exercise	Exercise Group	Set 1	Set 2	Set 3	Total	Progress
1	1	6/11/2020	Standard Push-Up	Push	9	8	6	23	
			Legs Straight Row	Pull	10	8	8	26	
			Standard Squat	Squat	12	12	11	35	
	2		Rest	Rest					
	3	6/13/2020	Standard Push-Up	Push	9	9	8	26	*
			Legs Straight Row	Pull	10	10	8	28	*
			Standard Squat	Squat	12	12	12	36	*
	4		Rest	Rest					
	5	6/15/2020	Standard Push-Up	Push	9	9	9	27	*
			Legs Straight Row	Pull	10	10	9	29	*
			Standard Squat	Squat	13	12	12	37	*
	6		Rest	Rest					
	7		Rest	Rest					

ADDITIONAL RESOURCES

Active stretching and warmup

https://www.youtube.com/watch?v=Tb_WdTCUCf8

Calisthenics exercise videos

https://www.youtube.com/user/sdrader/videos?view_as=subscriber

Grind-Style Calisthenics Explained

https://reddeltaproject.com/grind-style-calisthenics/

X+1 Rep Method

https://formiseverything.com/2020/03/27/introducing-the-x1-the-micro-workout-mini-measuring-stick/

The Form Is Everything Blog

https://formiseverything.com/blog/